Keto, Made Easy

Also by Kevin Klix:

FICTION

Biflocka
A Lion in Your Number
Elevator Music
Skateboy
The Student
Wasp in the Opium Flowers

NON-FICTION

Beautiful Nihilism
What's Wrong With Millennials?

SELF-HELP

A Wellness Guide to Happiness
Stop Unreality

POETRY

Why I F*cking Hate Poetry

Keto, Made Easy

The Clear-Cut Guide
to the Ketogenic Diet
for Busy Lives

Kevin Klix

k Publishing Co. | Est. 2012

DISCLAIMER

This book is for informational purposes only. The content is not intended to be a substitute for professional medical advice, diagnosis, or treatment. Always seek the advice of your physician or other qualified health providers with any questions you may have regarding a medical condition. The author and publisher are not responsible for any adverse effects or consequences resulting from the use of any suggestions, preparations, or procedures discussed in this book.

KETO, MADE EASY. Copyright © 2025 by Kevin Klix. All rights reserved. No part of this book may be reproduced, distributed, or transmitted in any form or by any means, including photocopying, recording, or other electronic or mechanical methods, without the prior written permission of the publisher, except in the case of brief quotations embodied in critical reviews and certain other non-commercial uses permitted by copyright law. For permission requests, please contact Permissions at kevinklix@yahoo.com.

Printed in the United States of America. This book is printed on acid-free recycled paper.

Follow the author on X (formally Twitter) and instagram: @kevinklix

FIRST EDITION

Interior and Cover Design by Kevin Klix

Text set in 10 pt. Minion Pro, Titles set to 35-10.5 pt. Hypatia Sans Pro

The e-book edition is available in Kindle, EPUB, and PDF formats.

Library of Congress Cataloguing-in-Publication Date is pending.

ISBN: 979-8-9907321-2-4 (paperback)
ISBN: 979-8-2309670-0-2 (digital)
ASIN: B0DPTGDWVG (Amazon e-book)

14 13 12 11 10 / 10 9 8 7 6 5 4 3 2 1

If you purchased this book without a cover, you should be aware that this book is stolen property. It was reported as "unsold and destroyed" to the publisher, and neither the author nor the publisher has received any payment for this "stripped book."

Dedication is given to Casey Milner-Knotts.

Weight loss has always been something both of us have struggled with, babe. I simply wanted to make this book for us to follow. Keto may not be right for everyone, but it surely is effective. . . .

And baby, I want to thank you for always pushing me to do better. You are the best. I love you so, so much. Enjoy!

CONTENTS

INTRODUCTION xi

CHAPTER ONE 15

WHY DO KETO?: THE RUNDOWN ON THE NEW AGE DIET SWEEPING THE NATION

CHAPTER TWO 21

IS KETO RIGHT FOR YOU?

CHAPTER THREE 30

GETTING STARTED: THE SHOPPING LIST, THE PREP, AND THE EXPECTATIONS

CHAPTER FOUR 37

THE DREADED KETO FLU: DEALING WITH THE SICKNESS THAT BEATS MOST

CHAPTER FIVE   44

THE FIRST TWO WEEKS: THE DISCOURAGING THOUGHTS, PUSHING THROUGH, MOTIVATING YOURSELF, AND HAVING PATIENCE

CHAPTER SIX   50

MAINTAINING KETO: THE AFTERMATH OF THE FIRST TWO WEEKS: KEEPING UP WITH YOUR TIMED GOAL

CHAPTER SEVEN   57

REACHING YOUR GOAL!: HOW TO CELEBRATE BY EASING YOURSELF BACK INTO CARBOHYDRATES

CHAPTER EIGHT   64

LIFE AND LIFESTYLE AFTER KETO: KEEPING THE WEIGHT OFF, EXERCISING, AND CHANGING YOUR DIET

CHAPTER NINE   71

BE KIND, AND REWIND?: COMING TO TERMS WITH ROADBLOCKS, RELAPSES IN WEIGHT, AND KETO REVAMPING

RECOMMENDED READING   78
FOOTNOTES   84

Keto, Made Easy

The Clear-Cut Guide to
the Ketogenic Diet for
Busy Lives

INTRODUCTION

I have always read books on Keto, but I was always left with a sense that maybe they over-explained things, or weren't as direct, or could have worded things much more simpler and straight-forwardly. Trimming the fat, as they say. . . .

That's exactly why I decided to write this book. I wanted to create something that cuts through the nonsense—a guide that is simple, practical, and approachable for anyone curious about Keto. Whether you're just starting out, looking for tips to make the lifestyle easier, or even if you've tried Keto before but felt overwhelmed—this book is for you.

Here, you won't find endless technical jargon or an overload of scientific details. Instead, I'll break things down into bite-sized, easy-to-digest pieces (pun intended) so you can focus on what really matters: Understanding how Keto works and making it work for *you*.

Think of this as your tiny 80-page Keto companion—something you can turn to for clarity, inspiration, and encouragement, without feeling like you're back in a chemistry class. My goal is to take the guesswork out of Keto and show you that it doesn't have to be complicated. In fact, it can be incredibly empowering, enjoyable, and transformative when you strip it down to its essentials.

When I first started my own Keto journey, I had all the same questions and frustrations that you might be feeling right now. What can I eat? Will I be hungry all the time? Is it sustainable? And perhaps the biggest one of all: Does it really work?

The truth is, Keto *does* work—but only if you approach it in a way that fits your life. That's one of the biggest lessons I've learned, and it's the driving force behind this book. Keto isn't a one-size-fits-all plan, and it doesn't have to be rigid or intimidating. Instead, it's a flexible framework that can be tailored to your goals, your preferences, and even your schedule.

In this book, I'll walk you through everything you need to know to succeed on Keto, without overwhelming you. You'll learn the core principles of the diet, how to adapt it to your lifestyle, and —perhaps most importantly—how to actually enjoy the process. Because let's face it: if you don't enjoy the journey, it's hard to stay on track. . . .

You have a busy life. You don't have hours to spend deciphering complicated concepts or flipping through endless pages looking for answers. That's why I've designed this book to work with your schedule, not against it.

Each chapter is written to stand on its own, so you can jump to whatever topic interests you most or revisit sections whenever you need a quick refresher. Whether you're meal prepping for the week, looking for motivation to stay on track, or troubleshooting a Keto challenge, this book will be there for you—clear, concise, and straight to the point.

To make things even easier, I've included tips, tricks, and highlights throughout the book. These are the nuggets of wisdom you can skim in seconds and apply right away. Think of them as your "cheat codes" for navigating Keto while juggling everything else life throws your way.

To keep things as clean and streamlined as possible, I've placed all the detailed references and footnotes at the very end of this book. This way, you won't get bogged down by technicalities or citations as you read, but you'll still have access to deeper information if you're curious. Think of it as an optional deep dive—available when you want it, but never in your way.

Remember, there's no perfect way to do Keto, and that's the beauty of it—it's flexible. The goal is progress, not perfection.

So, let's get started. Flip to the next page, or jump ahead to the part that speaks to you the most. This is your journey, and I'm here to help you every step of the way!

Enjoy. :)

Signed,
Kevin Klix
West Palm Beach, Florida
November 21st, 2024

CHAPTER ONE

WHY DO KETO?: THE RUNDOWN ON THE NEW AGE DIET SWEEPING THE NATION

The ketogenic diet—commonly known as "keto"—has taken the world by storm. You've likely seen it featured in magazines, heard about it from friends, or noticed the explosion of keto-friendly products lining the grocery store shelves. Even notable celebrity figures such as Halle Berry[1] and LeBron James[2] have publicly shared their use of keto for fitness and energy. But what exactly is all the hype about? Why has this diet, initially developed as a medical treatment for epilepsy,[3] become the go-to lifestyle for people seeking weight loss, mental clarity, and improved health?

Keto isn't just another fleeting diet trend. It's a scientifically-backed approach that focuses on drastically reducing carbohydrate intake and replacing it with fat. This shift in macronutrients pushes your body into a metabolic state called *ketosis*, where fat becomes your primary fuel source instead of glucose.[4] In ketosis, your body becomes highly efficient at burning fat for energy, which can lead to significant fat loss, steady energy levels, and even a reduction in appetite.

But why are so many people embracing keto over other diet trends? The answer lies in its simplicity, effectiveness, and the wide-ranging benefits it offers beyond just weight loss.

A Fat-Burning Machine

At its core, keto is about switching your body's fuel source. Normally, we burn glucose (from carbs) for energy. But when you severely limit carbs, your liver starts breaking down fat into molecules called *ketones*. These ketones replace glucose as your body's primary energy source, turning you into a fat-burning machine. This is why people on keto often see rapid fat loss—your body is literally burning through its fat stores to keep you going.

Steady Energy, No More Crashes

One of the biggest benefits of the keto diet is that it provides *stable energy* throughout the day.[5] By using fat and ketones for fuel, your body avoids the rollercoaster of blood sugar spikes and crashes that often come with high-carb diets. Many people on keto report feeling more alert, focused, and energetic—without that mid-afternoon slump.

Appetite Control: Say Goodbye to Hunger Pangs

Another reason keto stands out is its ability to curb appetite.[6] High-fat, low-carb meals keep you feeling full and satisfied for longer. This leads to less snacking and fewer cravings, which can make it easier to stick to the diet and reduce overall calorie intake. It's not just about restricting food—it's about retraining your body to rely on nutrient-dense, filling meals.

The Science Behind Keto's Health Benefits

The ketogenic diet, beyond just losing your gut's mass, has been linked to a wide range of health benefits. It has been shown to improve *heart health* by raising good HDL cholesterol and lowering triglycerides.[7] It can also enhance mental clarity and focus, as ketones provide an efficient energy source for the brain. Keto may even offer protection against certain diseases like Alzheimer's,[8] diabetes,[9] and some cancers,[10] by reducing inflammation and stabilizing blood sugar levels.

"But Isn't Eating Fat Bad?"

For decades, we've been told that fat is the enemy, most famously with the USDA Food Pyramid,[11] launched in 1992, that placed fats and oils at the very top, implying they should be used sparingly. Low-fat diets have been the standard prescription for weight loss and heart health. But in recent years, studies have called this conventional wisdom into question, such as into the DIETFITS study at Stanford University tested two diets—low-fat and low-carb—against each other in a weight loss and metabolic outcomes competition.[12] The results showed that both diets could be effective for weight loss, but neither proved superior across the board. While not all fats are created equal, the right fats—like those found in avocados, nuts, seeds, and olive oil—are essential for energy, cell function, and hormone regulation.

On the keto diet, the focus is on *healthy fats* & *whole foods* (refer to Chapter 3 for lists). When you remove processed carbs and sugars from your diet, you replace them with nutrient-dense fats and proteins, which can lead to a more balanced and sustainable way of eating.

Is Keto Right for You?

Keto isn't for everyone, but for many, it offers a sustainable, enjoyable way to eat. If you're looking for a way to shed fat, boost your energy, and regain control of your appetite, keto might be the solution you've been waiting for. But like any diet, it's important to understand how it fits into your lifestyle and health goals. Keto requires commitment, especially in the beginning, when your body is transitioning from burning carbs to burning fat. This process, often called the "keto flu," can come with some short-term side effects like fatigue, headaches, and irritability as your body adapts. However, once you've adjusted, many people find the long-term benefits far outweigh the temporary discomfort.

One of the key elements to succeeding on the ketogenic diet is planning. Because keto involves significantly reducing carbs and increasing fats, it requires a mindful approach to food choices. It's essential to make sure you're eating the right types of fats—those that are healthy and sustainable—while also ensuring that you're getting enough protein and avoiding hidden carbs that can throw you out of ketosis.

Why Keto Fits Busy Lives

A big part of keto's appeal, especially for people with hectic schedules, is its simplicity. Once you have a handle on the basic principles, keto doesn't require elaborate meal prepping or complicated recipes. You don't have to count calories meticulously. Instead, you focus on eating nutrient-dense, high-fat, low-carb foods that keep you satisfied for longer periods. This is why keto is particularly beneficial for people who want to avoid the constant cycle of snacking and hunger pangs.

For busy worker bees, mommas and papas, or anyone else juggling a packed schedule, keto can be streamlined into everyday life—and with ease. Meals can be as simple as a salad loaded with healthy fats like avocado and olive oil, or a quick stir-fry made with fatty cuts of meat and low-carb vegetables. The diet lends itself to quick, satisfying meals without the need to stress over complex cooking.

Beyond the Hype: Long-Term Keto Benefits

While keto has become trendy, its long-term benefits should not be overlooked. Unlike many crash diets, keto offers sustainable results by promoting a healthier relationship with food. By shifting away from sugar and processed carbs, you may find that your cravings diminish and your reliance on food for comfort or emotional eating decreases. For many, keto leads to a more mindful approach to eating, where food is seen as fuel rather than a source of indulgence or guilt.

Moreover, the long-term impact on overall health is promising. Keto's ability to reduce inflammation, regulate insulin levels, and promote fat loss has led to its increased use in therapeutic settings, helping individuals with conditions such as epilepsy, Type-2 diabetes, and metabolic syndrome. It's more than just a weight-loss plan; for many, it's a way of life that fosters better health and well-being.

The Next Step: What To Expect

Now that you have a general idea of what keto is and why it's gained such a dedicated following, the next part I would like to go over is deciding how keto—and all of its methods and quirks—can work for you. As you dive deeper into this book, you'll discover practical tips, meal plans, and strategies to make keto simple and accessible—even if you have a busy lifestyle, as the subtitle reads. Whether you're just curious about keto or ready to fully commit, this guide is designed to cut through the nonsense and give you the clear, actionable, bite-sized steps you need to succeed.

No fluff, no B.S.

Keto is more than just a diet. It's a shift in how you approach food, energy, and overall health. And while the road to ketosis might have its challenges, the rewards—sustained energy, fat loss, and mental clarity—are worth the journey. But please keep in mind that not all diets are created equal: people are entirely different and one diet may be right for one person and different for the other. Keto is just one of them. My purpose is to make sure that if you do try it, it is done precisely and with care and a good effort. Let's get started!

CHAPTER TWO

IS KETO RIGHT FOR YOU?

For you to understand whether the ketogenic diet is right for you, it's essential to grasp what happens behind the scenes when you shift from a carb-based metabolism to a fat-based one. . . . Unlike traditional diets that focus on restricting calories or specific food groups, keto takes a different approach: cut as much carbs as you can with the goal of *remaining in ketosis*. But not just carbs, you also have to look at how certain foods react inside the body and could possibly create glucose (sugar) under the radar. In short, keto is basic, and the process appears to be relatively seamless. . . .

Well . . . sort of.

Understanding Ketosis: the Metabolic Shift

Under normal circumstances, your body relies on glucose from carbohydrates as its primary source of energy. When you eat carbs—whether from bread, pasta, fruits, or sugary snacks—your digestive system breaks them down into glucose, which is then absorbed into your bloodstream and used by your cells for energy.

However, when you limit your carb intake to around 20-50 grams per day, your body has to find an alternative source of fuel.

With glucose no longer readily available, the body taps into its fat reserves and begins converting fat into molecules called *ketones*. This process takes place in the liver, and ketones become the new primary energy source for your body, especially for your brain, which typically relies heavily on glucose.

Only a few vegetables are not keto-friendly because of their higher content of carbs—especially starches—that, when digested, result in the production of glucose. Other examples of starchy vegetables include potatoes, sweet potatoes, and corn, which happen to contain a great level of starch. Starch is a complex carb that is easily digested into glucose upon consumption. Similar to that, parsnips and butternut squash happen to contain massive amounts of starch and sugar within them. A person then accounts for this when it gets converted into glucose, hence spiking the blood sugar and removing it from ketosis. While carrots and beets are not as starchy as potatoes, they generally do contain natural sugars that get converted into glucose, thus not being suitable if someone is on a strict keto diet. While peas are not as packed with starch, they carry a decent carb load and will raise blood sugar levels if portioning is larger than healthy. The glucose derived from the vegetables will make your body blind to entering or being in a state of ketosis, a metabolic state in which your body burns fat instead of glucose for fuel.

Carbohydrates: the Body's Default Fuel

Carbs are the body's preferred source of energy.[13] But you have to keep in mind that your body breaks them down into *glucose*, a simple sugar that is used to fuel everything from your muscles to your brain. Glucose is easily absorbed into the bloodstream, and once there, it's distributed to your cells to be burned for immediate energy.

But here's the catch: when you consume more carbs than your body needs for immediate energy, that excess glucose is stored as *glycogen* in your liver and muscles. Glycogen acts as a short-term energy reserve, ready to be converted back into glucose when your body needs it. However, the body can only store a limited amount of glycogen—once these stores are full, any excess glucose is converted into our dreaded fat cells.

On a traditional high-carb diet, your body constantly burns glucose for energy and stores the leftovers as fat. This is why carb-heavy diets often lead to weight gain—because once your glycogen stores are full, there's nowhere for the extra glucose to go but into fat cells. . . . Forget about the potential weight gain. When you rely on carbs for energy, there becomes a huge downside: *energy spikes and crashes*. Carbs, particularly simple sugars and refined carbs, cause rapid spikes in blood sugar, followed by a sharp drop as insulin works to bring glucose levels back down. This rollercoaster of energy highs and lows can leave you feeling sluggish, hungry, and craving more carbs throughout the day. . . . This will create a endless cycle in your daily life, leading to perpetually gaining weight or staying at your same undesired weight.

The Role of Glycogen: Short-Term Energy Storage

Glycogen plays an important role as a short-term energy buffer. When blood glucose levels drop—say, between meals or during exercise—your body taps into its glycogen stores to keep your energy levels stable. Your muscles and liver break down glycogen into glucose and release it into your bloodstream to be used for energy. . . . However, as mentioned earlier, your body's glycogen storage is limited. Once these reserves are depleted, your body needs to find a new energy source. This is where the ketogenic diet comes in.

What Happens to Blood Sugar and Insulin?

Another critical change that happens when you're in ketosis is the stabilization of blood sugar and insulin levels. On a typical high-carb diet, your blood sugar spikes after meals, causing your pancreas to release insulin to regulate glucose levels. High insulin levels promote fat storage, making it difficult to lose weight and leading to cravings and energy crashes throughout the day.

On keto, because you're eating very few carbs, your blood sugar levels remain stable, and insulin spikes are minimized. This stabilization of insulin makes it easier to burn fat and prevents the wild swings in hunger and energy that often accompany high-carb diets. For people with insulin resistance, pre-diabetes, or Type-2 diabetes, the keto diet can be particularly beneficial, as it helps restore proper insulin function and control blood sugar levels.[14]

Ketones: Fuel for Your Brain

One of the most surprising benefits of the ketogenic diet is its effect on brain function. Unlike other tissues in your body, your brain cannot run on fat directly. Instead, it typically relies on glucose. But in a state of ketosis, your brain adapts to using ketones as a primary energy source. Ketones are not only efficient fuel for your brain, but they also produce less oxidative stress and inflammation than glucose, leading to improved mental clarity, focus, and concentration. . . .

Reports of fewer brain fog moments and greater cognitive function while on keto is partly because ketones are a more stable and long-lasting energy source than glucose, which can fluctuate wildly depending on carb intake. The mental benefits of keto are one of the reasons it's being explored as a therapeutic diet for neurological conditions such as Alzheimer's disease and epilepsy.

What's Happening to Your Fat Stores?

One of the most noticeable effects of the ketogenic diet is the accelerated fat loss that happens when your body is in ketosis. Particularly around the abdominal area, which is associated with increased health risks like heart disease, type 2 diabetes, and metabolic syndrome. Excess abdominal fat, also known as visceral fat, surrounds vital organs and can lead to chronic inflammation, insulin resistance, and other serious health complications. So for those that look in the mirror and are dissatisfied with the size of your tummy, keto could make you see quick results.

In ketosis, your body also produces lower levels of insulin, which further encourages fat burning. High insulin levels are known to inhibit fat breakdown,[15] so reducing insulin through carb restriction opens the door for your body to tap into its fat reserves more easily.

Because fat and ketones provide a more stable energy supply than glucose, many people on keto experience a *reduced appetite*, which leads to fewer cravings and makes it easier to stick to the diet. This appetite suppression is a major reason why keto is effective for long-term weight management, as it helps people naturally reduce their caloric intake without feeling deprived.

Why Fat Is a More Efficient Fuel Source

One of the reasons keto is so effective is that *fat is a more efficient fuel source* than glucose. While glucose burns quickly and requires constant replenishment, fat burns more slowly and steadily, providing long-lasting energy.[16] This is why many people on keto report feeling more energetic and focused throughout the day—they're no longer riding the highs and lows of blood sugar fluctuations.

Fat is also a *more energy-dense macronutrient*. Each gram of fat provides 9 calories, compared to 4 calories per gram of carbs or protein. This means that fat is a more concentrated source of fuel, allowing your body to run on less food while still maintaining stable energy levels. And because your body can access its fat stores in ketosis, you're effectively turning your own body fat into energy, making keto a highly effective tool for fat loss.

Fats are more *satiating* than carbs, meaning they help you feel satisfied after meals and reduce the urge to overeat. Many people on keto find that they naturally consume fewer calories simply because they're not as hungry, which contributes to weight loss without the need for strict calorie counting.

The Role of Protein on Keto

While fat is the primary fuel source on keto, *protein* also plays an important role. Protein is essential for maintaining muscle mass, repairing tissues, and supporting various bodily functions. However, it's important to strike the right balance with protein intake on keto. . . . Too little protein can lead to muscle loss, especially if you're losing weight quickly. But too much protein can interfere with ketosis. When you consume excess protein, your body can convert it into glucose through a process called *gluconeogenesis*.[17] This glucose can then be used for energy, which may prevent your body from fully entering ketosis.

The key is to aim for *moderate protein intake*—enough to support muscle maintenance but not so much that it disrupts ketosis. Most people on keto aim for about 20-25% of their daily calories from protein, focusing on high-quality sources like meat, poultry, fish, eggs, and dairy.

The "Keto Flu": What To Expect During Your Transition

Circling back to my comment earlier in this chapter about keto being a "seamless process . . . sort of," I must warn you about the dreaded Keto Flu. While the keto diet offers many benefits, transitioning into ketosis isn't always easy on the body and mind. In the first few days or weeks of starting the diet, many people experience what's known as the "keto flu"—a group of symptoms that can include fatigue, headaches, irritability, and brain fog. These symptoms occur as your body adapts to burning fat instead of carbs . . . but they're usually temporary. . . .

The keto flu happens because your body is undergoing a major metabolic shift. During this transition, your body depletes its stored glycogen (the form of glucose stored in your muscles and liver), and with it, your body releases excess water and electrolytes. This can lead to dehydration and an imbalance in minerals like sodium, potassium, and magnesium.

To minimize the effects of the keto flu, it's important to stay hydrated, increase your intake of electrolytes, and give your body time to adjust. Once your body becomes fully adapted to using fat and ketones for fuel, these symptoms typically subside. . . . Most people who begin to feel the benefits of ketosis, such as increased energy and mental sharpness, start to understand just how severe a high sugar and carb-based diet have influenced their lives.

Is Keto Right for You, Though?

Now that we've explored what happens inside the body on keto, the next question is whether it is the right diet for you. . . . Keto can be a powerful tool for weight loss, managing blood sugar levels, and improving mental clarity, but it's not a one-size-fits-all solution.

Keto may be especially beneficial if you:

- **Struggle with blood sugar regulation:** If you have insulin resistance, pre-diabetes, or Type-2 diabetes, keto can help stabilize your blood sugar and improve insulin sensitivity.

- **Want sustainable fat loss:** For those looking to lose fat and keep it off, keto's fat-burning focus may provide long-term results.

- **Experience energy crashes or cravings:** If you find yourself constantly craving carbs or dealing with fluctuating energy levels, keto's steady energy supply may offer relief.

- **Need mental clarity:** Whether you're a student, professional, or simply want to optimize your cognitive function, keto's effect on brain health could help you feel sharper and more focused.

However, keto isn't for everyone. It may not be suitable for individuals with certain medical conditions such as liver or kidney issues, or for those who require higher carbohydrate intake for specific physical activities. As with any dietary change, it's important to consult with a healthcare professional before starting keto, especially if you have any underlying health concerns. . . .

The Bigger Picture: Metabolic Flexibility

One of the long-term benefits of keto is that it promotes *metabolic flexibility*—the ability to switch between using carbohydrates and fats for fuel. When you're on a high-carb diet, your body becomes dependent on glucose, making it difficult to burn fat efficiently. But once you're in ketosis, your body becomes more adept at using fat for energy, even if you occasionally consume carbs.

This metabolic flexibility can be a powerful tool for maintaining weight loss and overall health. It allows you to enjoy a wider range of foods while still tapping into the benefits of fat burning, reduced inflammation, and stable energy levels.

Mastering the Science Behind Keto

Understanding how carbs, glycogen, fats, and proteins interact with your body is the key to mastering the ketogenic diet. By limiting carbs, you force your body to switch from burning glucose to burning fat, which results in more efficient energy use, fat loss, and long-lasting satiety.

This metabolic shift is at the heart of why keto works. It's not just about what you eat—it's about retraining your body to use fat as its primary fuel source. With this knowledge in hand, you're better equipped to navigate the world of keto and make informed choices that will set you up for success.

In the next chapter, we'll dive into the practical steps of getting started on keto, including what to shop for, how to prepare, and what to expect in those crucial first few days. With a solid understanding of how keto affects your body, you'll be ready to begin your journey with complete confidence!

CHAPTER THREE

GETTING STARTED: THE SHOPPING LIST, THE PREP, AND THE EXPECTATIONS

Now that you understand the general science behind the ketogenic diet and how your body will react to it, it's time to dive into the practical side of things. Starting keto doesn't have to be complicated, but preparation is key to success. In this chapter, I will guide you through the essentials of getting started: a comprehensive shopping list, meal prepping strategies, and realistic expectations for what your first few days and weeks on keto might look like. The goal is to help you feel confident, organized, and ready to tackle keto with ease.

The Essential Keto Shopping List

The foundation of keto success is in the food you eat, and having the right ingredients on hand will make all the difference. I want to give you a keto-friendly shopping list designed to help you hit the ground running. The focus is on whole, unprocessed foods that are high in healthy fats, moderate in protein, and low in carbs.

Healthy Fats:

Fats are the cornerstone of the ketogenic diet. Stock up on a variety of healthy fats to fuel your body.

- ☐ Avocados
- ☐ Coconut oil
- ☐ Olive oil
- ☐ MCT oil
- ☐ Grass-fed butter or ghee
- ☐ Full-fat cream cheese
- ☐ Full-fat sour cream
- ☐ Heavy whipping cream
- ☐ Cheese (cheddar, mozzarella, gouda, etc.)
- ☐ Nuts & seeds (almonds, walnuts, chia seeds, flaxseeds)
- ☐ Nut butters (almond butter, peanut butter – no sugar)
- ☐ Mayonnaise (full-fat, sugar-free)

Protein Sources:

Moderate protein intake is key to keto. Focus on high-quality sources of protein that are low in carbs.

- ☐ Grass-fed beef
- ☐ Chicken thighs, drumsticks, and wings
- ☐ Pork chops, bacon, and sausage (sugar-free only)
- ☐ Fatty fish (salmon, mackerel, sardines)
- ☐ Eggs (organic or free-range if possible)
- ☐ Shellfish (shrimp, lobster, crab)
- ☐ Turkey
- ☐ Ground beef or ground turkey
- ☐ Tofu or tempeh (if vegetarian)

Low-Carb Vegetables:

Leafy greens and low-carb veggies are great for adding volume to your meals without spiking blood sugar.

- ❑ Spinach
- ❑ Kale
- ❑ Arugula
- ❑ Zucchini
- ❑ Broccoli
- ❑ Cauliflower
- ❑ Bell peppers (in moderation)
- ❑ Asparagus
- ❑ Cucumber
- ❑ Mushrooms
- ❑ Avocados (yes, they go here too!)
- ❑ Celery
- ❑ Lettuce (Romaine, butterhead, iceberg)
- ❑ Green beans

Keto-Friendly Fruits (in *strict* moderation):

While fruit should be limited on keto due to its sugar content, some low-carb fruits can be enjoyed—*in moderation!*

- ❑ Strawberries
- ❑ Blackberries
- ❑ Raspberries
- ❑ Lemons
- ❑ Limes
- ❑ Coconut (unsweetened)

Pantry Staples and Spices:

These staples will help you add flavor and variety to your keto meals.

- ☐ Salt (preferably Himalayan pink salt or sea salt)
- ☐ Black pepper
- ☐ Garlic powder
- ☐ Onion powder
- ☐ Paprika
- ☐ Italian seasoning
- ☐ Mustard
- ☐ Apple cider vinegar
- ☐ Sugar-free hot sauce (check labels)
- ☐ Soy sauce or coconut aminos (for a low-carb, soy-free option)
- ☐ Stevia or monk fruit sweetener (if you need a sugar substitute)

Having these staples on hand ensures you'll have the right ingredients to whip up keto-friendly meals without resorting to high-carb snacks or processed foods. By focusing on whole, nutrient-dense foods, you'll be setting yourself up for keto success from day one.

Meal Prepping for Success

Meal prepping is one of the best strategies to ensure you stay on track with keto, especially if you have a busy schedule. Prepping your meals in advance not only saves time, but it also reduces the temptation to reach for quick, carb-laden options when hunger strikes. Here's a simple plan to help you get started with keto meal prepping:

1. **Plan Your Week:**
   At the start of each week, take a few minutes to map out your meals. Decide on a few keto breakfast, lunch, and dinner options that you can rotate throughout the week. Include snacks if you think you'll need them.

2. **Batch Cook:**
   Choose a couple of keto-friendly recipes you can make in large quantities and store for later. For example, roast a large tray of chicken thighs and a big batch of roasted vegetables. These can be portioned out for multiple meals.

3. **Use Storage Containers:**
   Invest in high-quality food storage containers to portion out your meals. Glass containers are great because they can go straight from the fridge to the microwave. Having pre-portioned meals on hand makes it easy to grab and go, especially if you're heading to work or traveling.

4. **Prep Snacks:**
   Have keto-friendly snacks like boiled eggs, cheese sticks, nuts, and guacamole ready to go. Prepping your snacks ahead of time helps eliminate the urge to grab something carb-heavy when you need a quick energy boost.

5. **Keep it Simple:**
   Keto doesn't have to be complicated. Stick to simple meals that combine a healthy fat, a protein, and a low-carb vegetable. For example, grilled salmon with avocado and a side of sautéed spinach. The simpler the meal, the easier it is to stay on track.

Setting Expectations: the First Few Days and Weeks

Starting keto can feel like a big adjustment, and it's important to know what to expect. Your body is going through a significant metabolic shift, and that can come with some side effects. Setting realistic expectations for the first few days and weeks will help you stick with the plan and avoid discouragement.

The First Few Days:
During the first three to five days, your body is burning through its glycogen stores. As you deplete glycogen, your body starts adjusting to using fat for fuel. You might feel a little sluggish or tired during this transition—but that is completely normal. Your body is essentially retraining itself to burn fat for energy. . . .

The Keto Flu:
The keto flu happens because your body is losing electrolytes as it sheds water weight (stored glycogen holds water). Combat the keto flu by drinking plenty of water and replenishing your electrolytes with salt, magnesium, and potassium. . . .

Energy Levels Stabilize:
By the second week, most people begin to feel the benefits of keto. Your energy levels stabilize, and you'll experience fewer cravings for carbs. Many people report feeling more focused, mentally sharp, and energized once they're fully in ketosis. . . .

Fat Loss Begins:
The initial weight loss in the first week is often due to water weight, but as your body adapts to burning fat, you'll begin to see fat loss. Everyone's body responds differently, so be patient if the scale doesn't move immediately. Fat loss on keto tends to be steady and sustainable over time. . . .

Adjusting Your Mindset: Thinking of the Long-Term Benefits

Keto isn't a quick fix; it's a long-term lifestyle change. As you begin your keto journey, try to focus on the non-scale victories that come with the diet—things like improved energy, mental clarity, and reduced cravings. It's easy to get caught up in numbers on the scale, but true success on keto comes from how you feel and how well you're fueling your body.

Celebrate small milestones, and don't expect overnight transformation. Keto is a journey that requires time and patience, but with the right preparation and mindset, you'll see the benefits quickly unfold.

CHAPTER FOUR

THE DREADED KETO FLU: DEALING WITH THE SICKNESS THAT BEATS MOST

If you've ever heard people talk about the keto diet, there's one thing that almost always comes up: "THE KETO FLU." It sounds ominous, and for many, it's the most difficult hurdle when starting the ketogenic diet. But don't worry—it is temporary, manageable, and it will not last forever. The keto flu happens during your body's transition from burning carbs (glucose) for fuel to burning fat and ketones instead. While this transition is beneficial in the long run, it can feel like a rough patch as your body adjusts.

What Is the Keto Flu?

The keto flu isn't an actual virus or illness—it's the name given to the collection of symptoms some people experience when they first start a ketogenic diet. They're a result of your body's adjustment to using fat and ketones for energy instead of relying on carbs. Simply put: Keto Flu is the equivalent of a drug addict going through (mild) addiction withdraws. How bad the "withdraws" are depends on how much your previous diet before starting keto involved consuming carbs. . . .

Common symptoms of "the keto flu" include:

- Headaches
- Fatigue
- Irritability or mood swings
- Nausea
- Dizziness or lightheadedness
- Difficulty sleeping
- Muscle cramps or soreness
- Brain fog

As I've said, the symptoms of the keto flu can range from mild to more intense, depending on how dependent your body has been on carbs. For those who consumed a high-carb diet before starting keto, the transition can be a bit more challenging. But don't be discouraged—these symptoms are only temporary, and there are ways to manage them.

Why Does the Keto Flu Happen?

The keto flu is a natural consequence of your body switching its primary fuel source from carbs to fat. On a typical high-carb diet, your body burns glucose for energy. But when you drastically reduce your carbohydrate intake (usually to around 20-50 grams per day), your body has to find an alternative energy source. This is when it starts to burn fat for fuel and produces *ketones*.

During this metabolic shift, your body goes through several changes, including:

➡ **Depleted Glycogen Stores**: Glycogen, which is stored in your liver and muscles, is your body's reserve of glucose. When you stop eating carbs, your body begins to use up its glycogen stores. Since glycogen is stored with water, this depletion causes your body to lose water and electrolytes, which contributes to the symptoms of the keto flu.

➡ **Electrolyte Imbalance**: As your body flushes out water (often leading to initial weight loss), it also loses essential electrolytes like sodium, potassium, and magnesium. This imbalance can cause symptoms like headaches, fatigue, muscle cramps, and dizziness.

➡ **Reduced Insulin Levels**: On keto, your insulin levels drop because you're eating fewer carbs. While this is a good thing in the long term, as lower insulin promotes fat burning, it can also lead to a temporary imbalance in blood sugar, which contributes to feelings of tiredness, irritability, and brain fog.

➡ **Metabolic Shift**: The transition from burning glucose to burning fat is a major shift for your body. It takes time for your body to become efficient at producing and using ketones, which can leave you feeling sluggish and foggy in the beginning.

These changes are part of the body's adjustment to ketosis, and while they may be uncomfortable, they are *a sign that your body is making progress!*

How To Manage and Reduce Keto Flu Symptoms

Fortunately, the keto flu doesn't have to sideline your keto journey. With the right strategies, you can manage or even prevent many of the symptoms, making the transition smoother and much more manageable. Here's how to tackle the keto flu head-on:

Hydration Is Key

One of the most common causes of keto flu symptoms is *dehydration*. When you start keto, your body flushes out excess water as it depletes glycogen stores. To counteract this, make sure you're drinking *plenty of water*—aim for at least 8-10 glasses a day, and increase your intake if you're exercising or sweating.

Drinking enough water will help reduce symptoms like headaches, dizziness, and fatigue.[18] Staying hydrated also helps flush out any toxins that your body might be releasing as it adjusts to burning fat.[19]

Replenish Your Electrolytes

The loss of electrolytes—especially sodium, potassium, and magnesium—is a major contributor to keto flu symptoms. As your body sheds water, it also loses these essential minerals, leading to muscle cramps, headaches, and fatigue.

To combat this, make sure that you are replenishing your electrolytes throughout the day:

- **Sodium**: Add extra salt to your food or drink a cup of broth to boost your sodium intake. Himalayan pink salt or sea salt are excellent options.

- **Potassium**: Include potassium-rich foods like spinach, avocado, and mushrooms in your meals. You can also use a potassium supplement if needed.

- **Magnesium**: Consider taking a magnesium supplement, or add foods like almonds, leafy greens, and pumpkin seeds to your diet to ensure you're getting enough.

Replenishing these electrolytes will help balance your body's fluids and reduce symptoms like muscle cramps, headaches, and dizziness.

Eat Enough Fat

On keto, fat is your primary fuel source, so it is important to make sure you're eating enough of it. Many people new to keto make the mistake of cutting carbs but not increasing their fat intake enough, leaving their bodies without a sufficient energy source. This can make the keto flu worse, as your body struggles to find fuel.

Focus on eating healthy fats from sources like avocado, olive oil, coconut oil, butter, and fatty cuts of meat. Eating enough fat will help keep your energy levels steady and support the transition to fat burning.

Don't Skimp On Calories

While keto isn't about counting calories, it's important to ensure that you're eating enough food to fuel your body during this transition period. Cutting carbs too drastically or too quickly without increasing your fat and protein intake can lead to feelings of weakness, fatigue, and hunger.[20]

Listen to your body's hunger cues and make sure you're eating nutrient-dense meals that include healthy fats, moderate protein, and low-carb vegetables. Don't worry about restricting calories during this phase—focus on nourishing your body as it adapts to burning fat.

Ease Into Physical Activity

If you're feeling sluggish or fatigued during the first few days of keto, it's okay to take it easy with physical activity. Strenuous exercise can deplete your glycogen stores even faster, which may exacerbate keto flu symptoms. Focus on gentle, low-intensity activities like walking, stretching, or yoga until your energy levels return to normal.

Once your body has fully adapted to burning fat and you're feeling more energized, you can gradually increase the intensity of your workouts.

Get Plenty of Sleep

Your body is undergoing a significant metabolic shift, and adequate *rest* is crucial during this transition. Aim for at least 7-8 hours of quality sleep each night to support your body's adjustment to ketosis. Sleep will help reduce fatigue, improve mood, and boost overall recovery during the keto flu phase.

If you're struggling with sleep disturbances during this time (a common side effect), try implementing a calming bedtime routine, reducing screen time before bed, and keeping your sleep environment cool and comfortable.

Pushing Through: the Mental Game

The keto flu isn't just a physical challenge—it's a mental one, too. When you're dealing with fatigue, headaches, and cravings, it's easy to feel discouraged and wonder if keto is right for you—or is even working, or if it's even *going* to work. But it's important to remember that the keto flu is temporary, and the benefits that come after will be well worth the initial discomfort. I promise you.

Remind yourself that your body is doing hard work behind the scenes. The symptoms you're experiencing are a sign that you're depleting glycogen stores, stabilizing insulin levels, and making the shift toward fat burning. Once your body adapts to using fat and ketones for fuel, the *steady energy*, *mental clarity*, and *fat loss* will make all the effort worth it!

Surviving the Dreaded, Yucky Keto Flu!

The keto flu is a temporary phase that many people experience when starting the ketogenic diet, but it's manageable with the right strategies. By understanding why it happens and taking steps to replenish your body's hydration and electrolytes, you can ease the symptoms and make the transition to ketosis smoother. Keep in mind that the keto flu is just a *short-term hurdle* on the path to achieving long-term success on keto.

Once you push through this initial phase, your body will adjust, and the benefits will begin to shine. Stay patient, stay hydrated, and remember that the discomfort will pass. Your body is adapting to a new way of fueling itself, and soon enough, you'll be reaping the rewards of your hard work.... In the next chapter, we'll dive into what you can expect during *the first two weeks* of keto, including how to stay motivated, how to push through discouraging moments, and how to build momentum for long-term success.

CHAPTER FIVE

THE FIRST TWO WEEKS: THE DISCOURAGING THOUGHTS, PUSHING THROUGH, MOTIVATING YOURSELF, AND HAVING PATIENCE

The first two weeks of the ketogenic diet can be an emotional rollercoaster. You're excited to start your keto journey, yet after a few days, you might start questioning your decision. It's common to feel discouraged as your body adjusts, especially if cravings and discomfort set in. But know this: You are not alone! The first two weeks are often the most challenging part of keto, but they are also the most critical. If you can push through this initial phase, the benefits are well within reach.

The Mental Game: Why the First Two Weeks Are Tough

During these first two weeks, your body is learning how to efficiently produce and use ketones for fuel, and while this is happening, you may experience physical symptoms like fatigue, cravings, and brain fog. However, the *mental battle* is often the toughest part. You might find yourself asking: (1) "Why do I feel so tired? Is this diet really working?", (2) "Why am I craving carbs so badly?", and (3) "Should I just quit? This is harder than I thought."

These thoughts are normal, but they can make the process feel overwhelming. It's essential to recognize these feelings for what they are—a natural response to change. Remember, your body is adapting to a new way of eating, and with time, these challenges will pass. But first, let's talk about how to manage these discouraging thoughts and stay motivated.

Common Discouraging Thoughts (and How To Overcome Them)

1. **"I'm so tired—why isn't keto giving me energy yet?"**
   Fatigue is a common symptom in the early stages of keto. As your body depletes its glycogen stores and switches to burning fat, your energy levels might dip. This is especially true if you're experiencing *the keto flu* (as discussed in the previous chapter).
   How to overcome it: Stay hydrated, replenish your electrolytes, and give your body the time it needs to adjust. Many people notice a significant boost in energy after the first week or two. Remember, keto is about long-term results, not instant gratification.

2. **"I'm craving carbs so badly—maybe I should just eat a little bit of something sweet."**
   Cravings for carbs are a powerful mental hurdle. For many, carbs are a comfort food, and giving them up can feel like deprivation. These cravings are often strongest in the first week, as your body adjusts to lower glucose levels.
   How to overcome it: Focus on eating nutrient-dense meals that include plenty of healthy fats and moderate

protein to keep you full and satisfied. Cravings are often a sign that your body needs fuel, so make sure you're eating enough. If you do find yourself craving carbs, remind yourself that these feelings will *pass* as your body adapts to fat-burning.

3. **"I haven't lost weight yet—shouldn't keto work faster?"**
Many people expect immediate weight loss on keto, but the reality is that weight loss can vary from person to person. While some people lose water weight in the first week, others may not see significant changes until their body is fully adapted to ketosis. Fat loss takes time, and the scale is not always the best indicator of success in the early stages.
How to overcome it: Don't rely solely on the scale. Instead, focus on how you're feeling—are your energy levels stabilizing? Are your clothes fitting better? Are your cravings subsiding? These are all positive signs that keto is working, even if the scale doesn't immediately reflect it.

Pushing Through: Motivation and Strategies To Stay on Track

Pushing through the first two weeks requires a *combination of mental fortitude* and *practical strategies*. Here are some tips to help you stay motivated and committed, even when things get tough:

1. **Set Small, Achievable Goals**
It's easy to get overwhelmed if you're only focused on the end result. Instead, set *small, achievable goals* for yourself. These might include things like staying in ketosis for three days, meal prepping for the week, or getting through a social event without giving in to carb temptations. Each

time you hit one of these smaller milestones, take a moment to celebrate your progress. Every step counts!

2. **Plan Your Meals in Advance**
One of the best ways to stay motivated is to avoid the stress of making food decisions on the fly. Plan your meals for the week ahead, and prep as much as you can in advance. Knowing that you have delicious, keto-friendly meals ready to go will reduce the temptation to reach for non-keto foods and help you stay on track.

3. **Stay Connected to Your "Why"**
Remind yourself why you started keto in the first place. Whether it's for weight loss, improved energy, mental clarity, or better health, staying connected to your reason will help you push through tough moments. Write it down and keep it somewhere visible—on your fridge, your phone, or your desk—so you can easily reference it when doubts arise.

4. **Find a Support System**
Starting keto can feel isolating, especially if the people around you aren't on the same journey. Seek out support from friends, family, or online communities where you can connect with others who are experiencing the same challenges. Sharing your progress, setbacks, and triumphs with a supportive group can make a huge difference in staying motivated.

5. **Track Non-Scale Victories**
The scale doesn't always tell the full story, especially in the

first few weeks of keto. Instead of looking at the scale, focus on *non-scale victories* that reflect the positive changes happening in your body. These might include things like feeling more energized, sleeping better, noticing clearer skin, or fitting into your clothes more comfortably.

The Power of Patience: Trusting the Process

One of the most important things to remember during the first two weeks of keto is that *patience is key*. The ketogenic diet is a long-term lifestyle change, not a quick fix. It takes time for your body to fully adapt to burning fat and ketones for energy, and that adjustment period looks different for everyone.

Trust the process. Some people may feel the benefits of keto—like steady energy and reduced cravings—within the first week. For others, it may take a bit longer. But the results come when you stay consistent, patient, and focused on the bigger picture.

Remember, your body has likely been running on carbs for most of your life, so it's normal for the transition to take some time. The discomfort and cravings you feel now will eventually fade, giving way to the sustained energy, mental clarity, and fat loss that keto is known for.

Celebrating Small Milestones

During these first two weeks, it's important to recognize and celebrate the small milestones along the way. Every day that you stick to keto is a win, even if you don't see immediate results. Celebrate the fact that you're taking control of your health, learning about your body, and making positive changes.

Here are some small milestones worth celebrating:

- ★ Successfully completing a keto day without giving in to cravings.
- ★ Hitting your water and electrolyte goals for the day.
- ★ Prepping your meals for the week and staying on track.
- ★ Noticing *improved sleep* or energy levels, even if they're subtle.
- ★ Resisting temptation during a social event or gathering.

Each of these victories brings you one step closer to your long-term goals, and they deserve to be acknowledged and celebrated. Reward yourself with something non-food-related, like a new workout outfit, a relaxing day off, or a book you've been wanting to read.

Patience, Persistence, and Progress Are Everything

The first two weeks of keto are often the most challenging, but they are also the most crucial. If you can push through the discouraging thoughts, cravings, and fatigue, you'll set yourself up for long-term success. Stay patient with your body—it's going through a significant metabolic shift that takes time and persistence.

Celebrate your small milestones, stay connected to your reasons for starting, and remind yourself that the challenges you're facing are temporary. Soon, the benefits of keto will begin to reveal themselves, and you'll be glad you stayed the course! I promise you that! In the next chapter, we'll discuss how to maintain keto after the first two weeks, keeping up the momentum, and staying on track toward your health and wellness goals.

CHAPTER SIX

MAINTAINING KETO: THE AFTERMATH OF THE FIRST TWO WEEKS: KEEPING UP WITH YOUR TIMED GOAL

Congratulations! If you've made it through the first two weeks of keto, you've already achieved something great. By now, your body has likely started adjusting to ketosis, and you may have noticed some positive changes. But the real challenge of keto isn't just getting started—it's staying consistent and maintaining momentum over the long term.

Now that the initial adjustment period is behind you, this chapter will focus on how to keep up with your *timed goals*, stay consistent with your meal planning, and avoid slipping back into old habits. My goal here is to help you build keto into a sustainable lifestyle that aligns with your long-term health and wellness goals. . . .

Set Timed Goals for Long-Term Success

The best way to maintain keto after the first two weeks is by setting timed goals. These goals give you a clear direction and something to work toward, which can help prevent feelings of complacency. Setting specific, measurable, and achievable goals will keep you motivated and allow you to track your progress over time.

Start With a 30-Day Goal

If you've completed the first two weeks, try setting a 30-day goal. This could be something simple, like staying in ketosis for 30 consecutive days or reaching a specific fitness milestone while following keto. Having a concrete goal to work towards will keep you focused as you navigate the first month of keto.

Set Mid-Term Goals

Beyond 30 days, set mid-term goals, such as sticking to keto for 60 or 90 days. You can also focus on goals like achieving a certain weight loss target, hitting a fitness benchmark, or improving specific health metrics, like blood sugar or cholesterol levels. Mid-term goals give you something to aim for without feeling too far away.

Long-Term Vision

Long-term goals (6 months, 1 year, etc.) give you a broader vision for your health. These could include maintaining your weight loss, staying in ketosis for extended periods, or even transitioning into a more flexible version of keto that suits your lifestyle. Long-term goals help you see keto as more than just a diet—it is a radical lifestyle change!

The key to success is breaking down your overall keto journey into smaller, *achievable* milestones. This makes the process less overwhelming and gives you a sense of accomplishment as you progress. Be kind to yourself and your capabilities to prevent discouragement. Any small goal that is achieved is a win!

Stay Consistent With Meal Planning

You've likely developed a meal routine that works for you, but consistency is key for maintaining long-term success on keto. The temptation to fall back into old eating habits—especially carb-heavy ones—can be strong, particularly as time goes on. To stay on track, *meal planning* should continue to be a priority.

Keep Meal Prepping

Just as you did in the early days of keto, keep meal-prepping a part of your routine. Prepping meals ahead of time ensures you always have keto-friendly options on hand, reducing the temptation to grab convenience foods or make impulsive choices. Set aside one day a week (Sunday works well for many people) to plan your meals, grocery shop, and prep for the week ahead.

Rotate Go-to Meals

It's easy to fall into a rut of eating the same foods over and over, which can lead to boredom and cravings. Create a list of *go-to keto meals* that you love, and rotate them regularly to keep things fresh. Don't be afraid to try new recipes or experiment with different ingredients. Keto offers plenty of variety—take advantage of it!

Focus On Nutrient-Dense Foods

As you continue with keto, make sure your meals are packed with *nutrient-dense foods*. Focus on quality sources of fat (like avocados, olive oil, and fatty fish), moderate protein (like grass-fed beef, eggs, and poultry), and low-carb vegetables (like spinach, broccoli, and cauliflower). By eating nutrient-rich foods, you'll support your body's health and feel satisfied after meals, reducing the urge to stray from keto.

Avoid Keto-Treat Overload!

While keto-friendly treats and snacks can be a fun addition, be mindful not to rely too heavily on them. Products like keto cookies, cakes, and fat bombs should be enjoyed in moderation, as they can sometimes lead to cravings for more. Stick to whole, natural foods as much as possible for long-term success.

Beware of Complacency: Avoiding the "Comfort Zone"

Once you've experienced some success on keto, whether it's weight loss or improved energy, it can be easy to become complacent. This "comfort zone" can lead to slipping back into old habits or thinking that small cheats won't hurt your progress. While the occasional indulgence is normal, too many indulgences can stall your progress and make it harder to stay on track. Here's how to avoid slipping into complacency...

Stay Aware of "Carb Creep"

Carb creep happens when you gradually start consuming more carbohydrates without realizing it. Maybe you've added an extra serving of low-carb snacks or have been more lenient with portion sizes. Over time, these small additions can kick you out of ketosis. Stay mindful of your carb intake, and if you find yourself slipping, recheck your portions and food choices to ensure you're sticking to the plan.

Keep Your "Why" Front and Center

Just as you did when you first started keto, keep reminding yourself why you started in the first place. Whether your goal was to lose weight, improve your energy, or support your overall health, staying connected to your *why* will help you avoid falling into old habits. Write it down and revisit it when motivation dips.

Track Your Progress

It's easy to lose sight of how far you've come when you're focused on day-to-day decisions. Regularly track your progress—not just your weight, but also how you feel physically and mentally. Keeping a journal of your non-scale victories (such as improved sleep, better digestion, or increased energy) will keep you motivated to stick with keto for the long haul.

> ### Don't Overcomplicate It
>
> One of the most common mistakes people make is overcomplicating keto. You don't need elaborate meals or supplements to succeed. Stick to the basics: eat whole, high-fat, low-carb foods, stay hydrated, and keep your electrolytes balanced. Simplicity is often the key to consistency.

Stay Flexible and Adapt

While it's important to stay committed to keto, it's equally important to be *flexible* as life changes. Social events, holidays, travel, and other life circumstances can present challenges, but with the right strategies, you can maintain keto without feeling restricted.

> ### Plan Ahead for Social Events
>
> Attending a party or eating out at a restaurant doesn't have to throw you off track. Look at menus in advance, choose keto-friendly options, and don't be afraid to ask for substitutions. Bring your own keto dish to parties if needed, so you know there will be something you can eat.

> ### Be Kind to Yourself
>
> Slip-ups happen. Maybe you gave in to a craving, or maybe you overindulged at a holiday dinner. The key is to not let one small slip-up turn into a vicious spiral of bad decisions. Be kind to yourself, recognize that it is part of the journey. Always get back on track the next day.

Consider Carb Cycling

As you become more experienced with keto, you might want to experiment with *carb cycling*—incorporating higher-carb days periodically to replenish glycogen stores and give yourself a mental break from strict keto. Carb cycling can be especially beneficial for athletes or those who engage in high-intensity exercise. However, it's important to plan these higher-carb days carefully and ensure they don't derail your progress. . . .

Reassess and Adjust

Your needs and goals may change over time, so don't be afraid to adjust your approach to keto. Maybe your initial goal was to lose weight, but now you're more focused on maintaining your health & energy. Be open to reassessing your goals and making tweaks to your diet, as needed.

Consistency Is Key

Maintaining keto after the first two weeks is all about consistency, planning, and avoiding complacency. By setting *timed goals*, staying committed to meal prepping, and keeping an eye on your progress, you'll be able to maintain momentum and make keto a sustainable part of your lifestyle.

While challenges will arise—whether it's social events, cravings, or slip-ups—the key is to stay adaptable and remember that keto is a long-term investment in your health. As you continue on your keto journey, keep focusing on the bigger picture, celebrate milestones, and trust that the consistency you built will lead to lasting success!

CHAPTER SEVEN

REACHING YOUR GOAL!: HOW TO CELEBRATE BY EASING YOURSELF BACK INTO CARBOHYDRATES

You've worked hard, stayed disciplined, and now you've reached your specific keto goal. Reaching it is a huge milestone—and it's only natural to want to celebrate. But keep in mind that after months of careful carb restriction, you may wonder: *how can I celebrate without undoing all this grueling hard work?*

This chapter—arguably the most important—is all about celebrating your success while transitioning from strict keto back to a more balanced, sustainable diet—one that can incorporate carbs without compromising your progress. Whether you're looking to add carbs back into your diet long-term or just on holiday and special occasions, I'll cover how to do it *gradually* and *mindfully*, so you can enjoy your success without major setbacks.

Why Gradually Reintroduce Carbs?

After following keto for a significant amount of time, your body has adapted to burning fat and ketones for fuel. Introducing a large number of carbs all at once can be a shock to your system. Your body will rapidly produce insulin to deal with the sudden influx of glucose, which can lead to bloating, weight gain (mostly water weight), and even a return to sugar cravings.

That's why *gradual* reintroduction is key. Easing back into carbs will allow your body to adjust slowly, minimizing the risk of rapid weight gain and energy crashes. It's about finding a balance that works for you while still maintaining your progress. . . .

How to Gradually Reintroduce Carbs

Here are some steps to help you *ease back* into carbs while celebrating your success . . .

✓ **Start with Whole, Unprocessed Carbs**
  When reintroducing carbs, focus on *whole, unprocessed carbohydrates* that are nutrient-dense and low on the glycemic index. These carbs are less likely to cause blood sugar spikes and will provide more sustained energy. Great options include:

  o Sweet potatoes
  o Quinoa
  o Brown rice
  o Oats (steel-cut or rolled)
  o Legumes (lentils, chickpeas, black beans)
  o Fruits (berries, apples, pears, etc.)
  o Root vegetables (carrots, beets)

  Avoid refined sugars, white bread, and processed foods, as these can quickly lead to cravings and weight regain.

✓ **Start Small and Increase Slowly**
  Begin by adding *small amounts of carbs* into one or two meals

per day. You could start with 25-50 grams of carbs per day, depending on how strict your keto routine has been. Gradually increase your carb intake over time, allowing your body to adjust without feeling stressed or overwhelmed. . . . For example, add half a sweet potato or a serving of quinoa to your dinner. Then, over the course of a week or two, slowly increase your portion sizes or incorporate carbs into additional meals.

✓ **Monitor Your Body's Response**
As you reintroduce carbs, pay attention to how your body reacts. Are you feeling more energized, or are you experiencing blood sugar crashes? Are cravings returning, or are you able to maintain balance? Tracking your energy levels, mood, and appetite will help you determine the right amount of carbs for your body. . . . Everyone's tolerance for carbs is different, so it's important to listen to your body and adjust accordingly.

✓ **Stay Mindful of Portions**
One of the biggest challenges in reintroducing carbs is staying mindful of *portion sizes*. After being on keto, it's easy to overestimate how many carbs you can handle without disrupting your progress. Stick to small portions in the beginning, and be aware of how those carbs affect your hunger and energy levels. . . . If you find yourself feeling sluggish or craving more carbs, it's a sign that you may need to dial back and reintroduce carbs more slowly.

Carb Cycling: a Balanced Approach to Reintroduction

One strategy for incorporating carbs while still maintaining the benefits of keto is *carb cycling*. This approach involves alternating between days of higher carb intake and days of low-carb or keto eating. Carb cycling can provide a mental break from strict keto, while also helping replenish glycogen stores and supporting workouts or physical activity.

> **Low-Carb Days**
>
> On low-carb days, stick to your typical ketogenic eating pattern—focusing on healthy fats, moderate protein, and minimal carbs (usually 20-50 grams per day). These low-carb days help you stay in ketosis and continue burning fat for energy. . . .

> **High-Carb Days**
>
> On high-carb days, increase your carbohydrate intake to around 100-150 grams. Focus on whole, unprocessed carbs, like sweet potatoes, quinoa, or oats. High-carb days are ideal for days when you're more physically active, such as workout days or days when you need extra energy.
>
> By alternating between low-carb and high-carb days, you can enjoy the benefits of both ketosis and the flexibility of including carbs in your diet. Carb cycling allows you to maintain balance and avoid falling back into old habits of carb-heavy eating.

How To Avoid Regaining Weight

One of the biggest fears people have after reaching their keto goal is regaining the weight they worked so hard to lose. It's obviously a valid concern, especially if you're starting carb-use again. Strategizing is key to not gaining or losing progress.

✓ **Prioritize Protein and Fiber**
As you reintroduce carbs, continue to prioritize *protein* and *fiber* in your meals. Protein helps keep you full and supports muscle maintenance, while fiber slows down the digestion of carbs, preventing blood sugar spikes. This combination will help you feel satisfied while keeping your appetite and cravings in check.

✓ **Stay Active**
Physical activity plays a crucial role in maintaining your weight, especially when you start eating more carbs. Regular exercise helps burn off extra glycogen, prevents weight gain, and improves insulin sensitivity. Incorporate a mix of strength training, cardio, and low-intensity activities like walking to support your health.

✓ **Mind Your Cravings**
Carbs, especially sugary and processed ones, can trigger cravings and lead to overeating. Stay mindful of the types of carbs you're consuming. If you notice that certain foods are triggering cravings (like refined carbs or sugary treats), scale back and focus on whole, nutrient-dense carbs instead.

✓ **Continue Intermittent Fasting (Completely Optional)**
If you've been practicing *intermittent fasting* during keto, please consider continuing this habit as you reintroduce carbs. Fasting helps control hunger hormones, supports fat loss, and stabilizes blood sugar. You don't have to fast every day, but incorporating intermittent fasting a few times a week can help maintain your results.

✓ **Don't Rush the Process**
The key to successfully reintroducing carbs without weight gain is to *take it slow!* Gradually increasing your carb intake over several weeks or months will give your body time to adjust. Rushing back into a high-carb diet is a surefire way to regain weight and derail your progress.

Enjoying Your Success Without Major Setbacks

Reaching your keto goal is something to celebrate, but the celebration doesn't have to involve undoing all of your hard work. There are plenty of ways to enjoy your success while maintaining the balance you've achieved through keto . . .

✓ **Celebrate with Non-Food Rewards**
Instead of celebrating your success with carb-heavy or sugary foods, find non-food rewards that align with your healthy lifestyle. Treat yourself to new workout gear, book a relaxing massage, or plan a fun day out with friends!

✓ **Mindfully Enjoy Occasional Indulgences**
If you do choose to celebrate with food, do it mindfully. Enjoy a slice of cake or a small serving of pasta without guilt, but keep it within moderation. Savor the experience and remind yourself that this is a special occasion, not a return to old habits. You only live once, as they say. . . .

✓ **Stay Focused on Long-Term Health**
Now that you've reached your goal, it's important to shift your focus from short-term achievements to *long-term health*. Instead of seeing your goal as the finish line, view it as the start of a new chapter where you continue to prioritize your well-being, make mindful food choices, and stay active.

A Balanced Path Forward

Reaching your keto goal is an incredible achievement, and you deserve to celebrate it. But as you ease back into using carbs again, it is important to do so gradually and mindfully. By focusing on whole, unprocessed carbs, staying active, and keeping an eye on your body's response, you can maintain your progress without major setbacks.

Whether you choose to transition into a balanced diet or experiment with carb cycling, remember that the key to success is *balance*. Keto doesn't have to be an all-or-nothing approach. It's about finding what works best for you, maintaining your results, and enjoying the benefits of a healthy, sustainable lifestyle.

CHAPTER EIGHT

LIFE AND LIFESTYLE AFTER KETO: KEEPING THE WEIGHT OFF, EXERCISING, AND CHANGING YOUR DIET

Reaching your goals is a major accomplishment, but the real journey begins once you transition to *life after keto*. You have worked really hard to lose weight, improve your health, and gain more energy—now the focus needs to shift into maintaining those results over the long haul. . . .

Maintaining Weight Loss: the Post-Keto Approach

The key to maintaining weight loss after keto is *balance*. Keto has helped you reach your goals by training your body to burn fat efficiently, but life doesn't have to be restricted to low-carb eating forever and ever. The transition to post-keto life involves finding a healthy equilibrium that works for you—a diet that allows for flexibility, enjoyment, and long-term health.

✓ **Continue Prioritizing Protein and Healthy Fats**
Even after keto, protein and healthy fats should remain the foundation of your meals. Protein helps you feel full and

satisfied, supports muscle maintenance, and keeps your metabolism active. Healthy fats provide long-lasting energy and help regulate hormones.

Build your meals around protein sources like chicken, fish, eggs, and lean meats, and incorporate fats from avocado, olive oil, nuts, and seeds. These macronutrients will help keep you satisfied and prevent overeating, even as you gradually reintroduce carbs into your diet.

✓ **Be Mindful of the Carbs You Ingest**

As you transition from keto, you don't need to avoid carbs entirely—but be mindful of your carb choices. Focus on whole, unprocessed carbs that are rich in fiber and low on the glycemic index so your blood sugar doesn't spike.

Pay attention to how your body responds to different carbs and adjust accordingly. You may find that your tolerance for carbs has changed after keto, and you'll need to experiment with portion sizes to maintain your results and feel okay.

✓ **Practice Mindful Eating**

After keto, it is easy to slip back into old habits of mindless snacking or emotional eating. But mindful eating is one of the most powerful tools for maintaining weight loss. Pay attention to your hunger and fullness cues, savor your meals, and avoid eating out of boredom or stress. This will help prevent overeating and keep you connected to your body's needs.

The Role of Exercise in Sustaining Progress

While keto helps you shed fat and improve your health, exercise is essential for maintaining those results and promoting overall well-being. Regular physical activity boosts your metabolism,[21] preserves muscle mass,[22] and enhances fat loss,[23] making it a crucial part of your post-keto lifestyle.

Strength Training for Muscle Maintenance

Strength training is one of the most effective forms of exercise for maintaining weight loss. Building and maintaining muscle mass increases your resting metabolic rate, meaning you burn more calories even when you're not exercising. Incorporating weight lifting, resistance training, or bodyweight exercises 2-3 times a week will help you stay lean and strong.

Cardio for Heart Health and Fat Loss

Cardiovascular exercise is important for heart health and fat loss. Whether it's walking, jogging, cycling, or swimming, aim for at least 150 minutes of moderate-intensity cardio each week. Cardio helps burn calories and improves your endurance, supporting your overall fitness and helping maintain your weight loss.

Stay Active Throughout the Day

While structured workouts are important, staying active throughout the day is just as crucial for maintaining your results. Incorporate movement into your daily routine by taking walks, standing instead of sitting, or doing stretches during breaks. These small actions add up and help you stay fit in the long run.

> **Focus on Consistency, Not Perfection**
>
> You don't need to be perfect with your workouts—consistency is the key to success. Find activities you enjoy and stick with them. The goal is to make exercise a regular part of your life, rather than a temporary fix. Whether it's yoga, hiking, dancing, or going to the gym, choose activities that keep you motivated and engaged.

Creating a Flexible, Sustainable Diet

As you move beyond keto, the goal is to create a flexible diet that aligns with your long-term health goals outside of keto itself. A balanced approach to eating allows you to enjoy a wider variety of foods while still maintaining the principles that helped you succeed on keto.

✓ **Embrace a Balanced Plate**
A well-balanced plate includes healthy fats, moderate protein, and whole carbs. Think of your meals as 50% non-starchy vegetables, 25% protein, and 25% healthy carbs or fats. This approach ensures you're getting the nutrients your body needs without overloading on any one macronutrient.

✓ **Continue Focusing on Whole Foods**
The success of keto is built on eating whole, nutrient-dense foods, and that shouldn't change after keto. Continue focusing on whole foods like vegetables, lean meats, fish, nuts, seeds, and healthy fats. Avoid processed, sugary, and refined foods, as they can lead to cravings and weight regain.

✓ **Don't Fear Carbs—But Choose Wisely**
Carbs are not the enemy, but it's important to choose the right ones.

✓ **Enjoy Flexibility with Occasional Treats**
After months of following keto, it's okay to enjoy occasional treats—but moderation is key. If you have a special event, holiday, or celebration, don't feel guilty about indulging. Just remember to return to your balanced eating plan afterward.

Avoiding the Slippery Slope

As you transition to life after keto, it's important to remain mindful of the old habits that can creep back in—habits like emotional eating, mindless snacking, or turning to food for comfort. Being aware of these patterns will help you prevent setbacks and stay on track.

Check-in With Yourself Regularly

Periodically check in with yourself to assess how you're feeling physically and emotionally. Are you still feeling energized? Are you relying on food to cope with stress? These check-ins help you stay connected to your body's needs and prevent slipping into old habits.

Stay Consistent With Meal Planning

Even after keto, meal planning is one of the best ways to maintain control over your diet. Plan your meals for the week ahead, stock your kitchen with healthy ingredients, and continue prepping meals in advance. This reduces the temptation to rely on takeout or processed foods.

> ### Don't Let Setbacks Spiral You
>
> Everyone has setbacks from time to time, whether it's overeating at a holiday meal or indulging in sugary treats. The key is to not let one setback turn into a spiral. If you slip up, acknowledge it, and then get right back on track with your next meal. Consistency over time is what matters most.

The Shift From Keto to Long-Term Health

Keto helped you reach your goals, but now it's time to focus on maintaining those results through long-term health. A healthy, balanced lifestyle goes beyond just simply macronutrients, et cetera—it is about nourishing your body with whole foods, staying active, and managing stress.

- ✓ **Prioritize Gut Health**
  Gut health is key to overall well-being. Incorporate fermented foods like yogurt, sauerkraut, and kimchi into your diet to support a healthy gut microbiome. Probiotics and fiber-rich foods also promote gut health, aiding digestion and supporting your immune system.

- ✓ **Stay Hydrated**
  Hydration is just as important after keto as it was during. Make sure you're drinking enough water each day to support digestion, energy levels, and overall health. Herbal teas and infused water can add variety to your hydration routine.

- ✓ **Manage Stress**
  Chronic stress can derail your health goals and lead to emotional eating, weight gain, and fatigue. Incorporate

stress-reduction techniques into your daily life, such as meditation, deep breathing, or mindfulness practices. Managing stress helps you stay grounded and focused on your health.

✓ **Prioritize Sleep**
Sleep is essential for maintaining your weight and overall health. Aim for 7 to 8 hours of quality sleep each night to support your metabolism, energy levels, and immune system. . . .

Building a Healthy, Sustainable Lifestyle

Life after keto is all about maintaining the progress you've made while embracing a flexible, balanced lifestyle that supports your health for the long term. By continuing to prioritize nutrient-dense foods, staying active, and being mindful of your habits, you'll be able to enjoy the benefits of keto without feeling restricted or deprived.

Remember, keto is just one tool in your health toolbox. As you transition into a more varied diet, focus on building a sustainable lifestyle that aligns with your goals, supports your well-being, and allows you to enjoy life to the fullest. You can always make your best judgement when it comes to these sorts of things. If it doesn't feel right to do, don't do it. Always do your best to remain responsible, as well as making sure you are held accountable.

CHAPTER NINE

BE KIND, AND REWIND?: COMING TO TERMS WITH ROADBLOCKS, RELAPSES IN WEIGHT, AND KETO REVAMPING

If there is one thing to remember as you move forward in your health journey, it's this: setbacks are normal. Whether it's a few pounds regained after a holiday, a lapse in consistency, or a stressful life event that throws your routine off course, these moments are part of the process. And here's the truth—they don't define your success.

Roadblocks and *relapses*—those times when things don't go exactly as planned. Maybe you've hit a weight plateau, maybe you've found yourself eating your favorite unhealthy food daily . . . or maybe life got in the way, and keto took a back seat. . . . Whatever the case may be, it is important to approach these moments with kindness, understanding, and the knowledge that you can always get back on track. Keto will always work for you when you know it worked for you in the past. Its your body and mind are ready for the task. *Progress is not linear*—but with the right mindset, you can continue moving forward. . . .

Weight Regain

Weight fluctuations are a normal part of any health journey, and a few pounds regained doesn't erase the progress you've made. Water retention, stress, or changes in your diet can all cause weight to fluctuate. Don't let a temporary setback make you feel like you've failed—view it as part of your journey and use it as a learning experience.

Stalled Progress or Plateaus

Hitting a weight loss plateau can be frustrating. After seeing steady progress, it may seem like your body is suddenly refusing to cooperate. . . . Plateaus are common, especially after significant weight loss. Your body may need time to adjust before continuing to shed fat. Patience is the soul virtue in keto—your progress hasn't stopped, even if the scale isn't moving.

Life Events and Stress

Life happens. Whether it's a family emergency, a new job, or a stressful period, it is normal to have moments where your keto routine takes a back seat. Don't be hard on yourself—these are times when you need to be kind to yourself and acknowledge that life is about balance. What is important is how you respond once things settle down.

Relapses Are Part of the Journey

The first thing to understand about relapses is that they're not the end of your keto journey—they're simply a detour. You might fall off the wagon temporarily, but that doesn't mean you've lost all the progress you've made. In fact, these moments can serve as valuable lessons, helping you refine your approach and strengthen your commitment.

✓ **Don't Dwell on the Past**
When you experience a setback, it's easy to get stuck in a cycle of guilt or disappointment. But the truth is, dwelling on the past won't change it. . . . Always make sure that you focus on what you *can* do today to always get back on track! Whether that means preparing a healthy keto meal, taking a walk, or simply drinking more water, every small action actually does count.

✓ **Remember Why You Started**
When you feel discouraged, remind yourself of the reasons you started keto in the first place. Was it to lose weight, gain energy, improve your health, or feel more confident? Reconnecting with your "why" will reignite your motivation and help you move forward with a renewed sense of purpose.

✓ **Reflect on What Worked and What Didn't**
Setbacks often offer valuable insights. Take a moment to reflect on what led to the relapse—was it stress, convenience, or cravings? By identifying the triggers, you can develop a strategy to prevent similar setbacks in the future. This isn't about blaming yourself—it's about learning and growing.

Redoing Keto: Getting Back on Track

The beauty of keto is that you can always restart. If you've fallen off track, don't be afraid to hit the reset button and get back to the basics. Whether it's a full reboot or a minor adjustment, getting back into ketosis is completely doable.

✓ Go Back to Keto Basics
Sometimes, the best way to get back on track is to simplify. Go back to the keto fundamentals—focus on eating whole, unprocessed foods, healthy fats, moderate protein, and low-carb vegetables. Plan your meals in advance, and avoid processed keto snacks that can derail your progress. Starting fresh with the basics will help your body transition back into ketosis smoothly.

✓ Ease Back Into Ketosis
If you've been out of ketosis for a while, remember that your body will need time to adjust as it re-enters ketosis. You might experience some *mild keto flu symptoms*, but they will pass as your body shifts back to fat burning. Stay hydrated, replenish electrolytes, and be patient with the process.

✓ Set Short-Term Goals
Aim to stay in ketosis for one week, or focus on drinking a certain amount of water each day. These small goals build momentum and give you a sense of accomplishment as you work your way back to where you want to be.

✓ Stay Kind to Yourself
It's easy to be hard on yourself after a setback, but self-compassion is key to success. Treat yourself with kindness

and remember that everyone experiences ups and downs. Your keto journey is unique to you, and it's okay to take a step back before moving forward again.

Maintaining a Positive Mindset

One of the most important factors in long-term success—whether on keto or any lifestyle change—is maintaining a *positive mindset*. Setbacks don't define you, and they certainly don't mean failure.

✓ **Celebrate Your Progress**
Focus on how far you've come rather than how far you have to go. Celebrate the victories—big and small—along the way. Whether it's losing weight, feeling more energetic, or having better mental clarity, acknowledging these successes will help you stay motivated, even during challenging times.

✓ **Surround Yourself with Support**
A strong support system can make all the difference in maintaining a positive outlook. Whether it's family, friends, or an online keto community, connecting with others who share your same goals will provide encouragement and accountability. Don't be afraid to ask for support when you need it.

✓ **Practice Gratitude**
A daily *gratitude practice* can help shift your focus from setbacks to the positive aspects of your journey. Take a few moments each day to reflect on what you're grateful for—whether it is your health, your progress, or simply the fact that you're committed to improving your well-being. Gratitude helps keep setbacks in perspective and reminds you of the bigger picture.

✓ **Reframe Setbacks as Learning Opportunities**
Rather than viewing setbacks as failures, see them as *learning opportunities*. What can you take away from the experience? How can you adjust your approach moving forward? This mindset shift allows you to grow from setbacks and become even more resilient in the face of future challenges.

The Power of Persistence

Like most things that are difficult in life, keto is not a sprint—it's a journey that requires *persistence* and patience. There will be ups and downs, but what matters most is your ability to keep moving forward and snapping back onto your desired path. Every day is a new opportunity to make choices that align with your health goals, and every small victory brings you closer to long-term success.

Remember, the road to health is not a straight line. There will be detours—and that's perfectly okay! What defines your journey is not perfection but your ability to persevere, learn from setbacks, and stay committed to your well-being.

Progress, Not Perfection

As we come to the end of this book, I want to leave you with this: *progress, not perfection*. Keto, like any lifestyle change, is about creating positive habits and making choices that support your health. There will be roadblocks and setbacks along the way, but these are simply part of the journey. Keto is a tool meant to teach you about how food reacts with your body and mind.

The fact that you're here—reading, learning, and committed to your health—means you've already made incredible progress. Be kind to yourself, celebrate your successes, and remember that you can always get back on track. Whether you need to restart keto, adjust your approach, or simply stay the course, know that you have the tools, the knowledge, and the resilience to succeed. I hope this book was simple enough and concise enough to give you some peace of mind, the tools, and the education in order to succeed and reach your health goals.

Every step you take is a step toward a healthier, happier you. Keep moving forward, stay positive, and embrace the journey—you're already winning! :)

RECOMMENDED READING

- **The Keto Reset Diet** by Mark Sisson
  Reboot Your Metabolism in 21 Days and Burn Fat Forever.

- **The Art and Science of Low Carbohydrate Living** by Dr. Jeff Volek and Dr. Stephen Phinney
  An Expert Guide to Making the Life-Saving Benefits of Carbohydrate Restriction Sustainable and Enjoyable.

- **The Complete Guide to Fasting** by Dr. Jason Fung
  Heal Your Body Through Intermittent, Alternate-Day, and Extended Fasting.

- **The Keto Diet: The Complete Guide to a High-Fat Diet** by Leanne Vogel
  Includes More Than 125 Delectable Recipes and 5 Meal Plans to Shed Weight, Heal Your Body, and Regain Confidence.

- **Good Calories, Bad Calories** by Gary Taubes
  Fats, Carbs, and the Controversial Science of Diet and Health.

- **The Case Against Sugar** by Gary Taubes
  A Deep Dive into the Health Consequences of Sugar and Its Role in Modern Diets.

- **Why We Get Fat: And What to Do About It** by Gary Taubes
  Explains the science of fat accumulation and offers solutions for effective weight management.

- **The Big Fat Surprise** by Nina Teicholz
  Why Butter, Meat, and Cheese Belong in a Healthy Diet.

- **Keto Clarity** by Jimmy Moore and Dr. Eric Westman
  Your Definitive Guide to the Benefits of a Low-Carb, High-Fat Diet.

- **The Obesity Code** by Dr. Jason Fung
  Unlocking the Secrets of Weight Loss through a Hormonal Approach.

- **Grain Brain** by Dr. David Perlmutter
  The Surprising Truth About Wheat, Carbs, and Sugar—Your Brain's Silent Killers.

- **Primal Blueprint** by Mark Sisson
  Reprogram Your Genes for Effortless Weight Loss, Vibrant Health, and Boundless Energy.

- **Real Food Keto** by Jimmy Moore and Christine Moore
  Applying Nutritional Therapy to Your Low-Carb, High-Fat Diet.

- **Eat Fat, Get Thin** by Dr. Mark Hyman
  Why the Fat We Eat Is the Key to Sustained Weight Loss and Vibrant Health.

- **The Keto Reset Instant Pot Cookbook** by Mark Sisson and Lindsay Taylor
  Reboot Your Metabolism with Simple, Keto-Friendly Recipes.

Did you enjoy this book?!

Please, if you would kindly go online to . . .

✓   www.goodreads.com

✓   www.amazon.com

Search the title of this book and please take a second to post an honest review! Tell other readers what you thought of it!

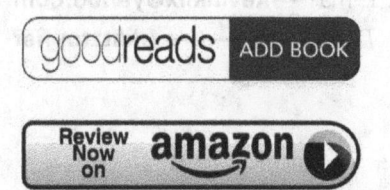

AUTHOR CONTACT INFORMATION

Instagram ——— **@kevinklix**
X, formally *Twitter* —— **@kevinklix**
E-mail — **kevinklix@yahoo.com**
TikTok ———— **@klitztopher**

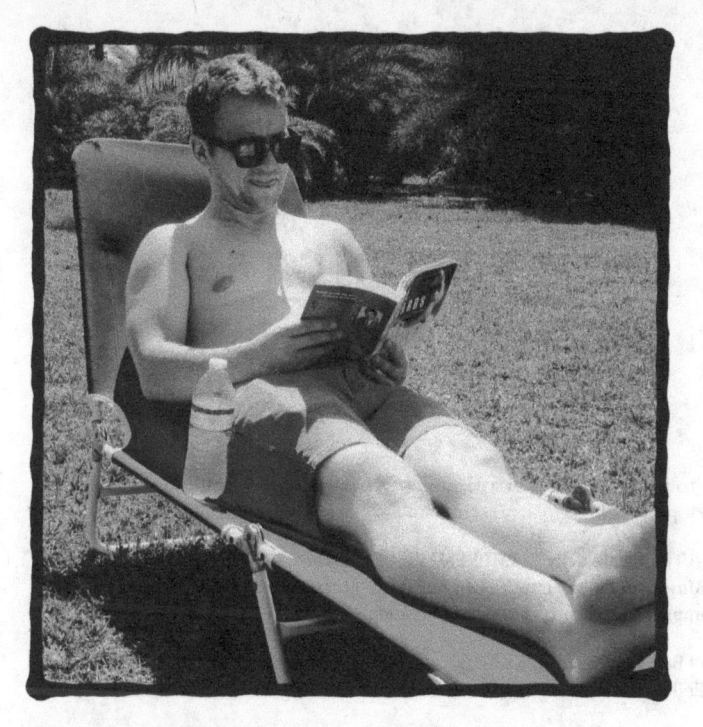

PHOTO BY CASEY MILNER-KNOTTS

About the Author:

Kevin Klix lives and works in West Palm Beach, Florida, with his girlfriend, Casey, and his dog, Pip. He has written six novels, two self-helps, three non-fiction works, and one collection of poetry. He enjoys writing on his typewriter and frequently posts poetry on his Instagram account (@kevinklix). In his free time, he does ink drawings, practices digital and film photography, and plays Blues on his electric guitar.

FOOTNOTES

[1] Stern, Abby. "Halle Berry Explains What She Eats to 'Live the Keto Lifestyle'". *People.com*. https://people.com/food/halle-berry-ketogentic-diet/

[2] Twardziak, Kelly. "8 IMPRESSIVE CELEBRITY KETO TRANSFORMATIONS". *Muscles & Fitness*. https://www.muscleandfitness.com/athletes-celebrities/news/8-impressive-celebrity-keto-transformations/

[3] Borowicz-Reutt K, Krawczyk M, Czernia J. Ketogenic Diet in the Treatment of Epilepsy. *Nutrients*. 2024; 16(9):1258. https://doi.org/10.3390/nu16091258

[4] Cleveland Clinic Staff. "Ketosis". *Cleveland Clinic*. https://my.clevelandclinic.org/health/articles/24003-ketosis

[5] Urbain, P., Strom, L., Morawski, L. *et al*. Impact of a 6-week non-energy-restricted ketogenic diet on physical fitness, body composition and biochemical parameters in healthy adults. *Nutr Metab (Lond)* 14, 17 (2017). https://doi.org/10.1186/s12986-017-0175-5

[6] Batch JT, Lamsal SP, Adkins M, Sultan S, Ramirez MN. Advantages and Disadvantages of the Ketogenic Diet: A Review Article. Cureus. 2020 Aug 10;12(8):e9639. doi: 10.7759/cureus.9639. PMID: 32923239; PMCID: PMC7480775.

[7] Sharman, M., Kraemer, W., Love, D., Avery, N., Gómez, A., Scheett, T., & Volek, J. (2002). A ketogenic diet favorably affects serum biomarkers for cardiovascular disease in normal-weight men.. *The Journal of nutrition*, 132 7, 1879-85 . https://doi.org/10.1093/JN/132.7.1879.

[8] Rusek, M., Pluta, R., Ułamek-Kozioł, M., & Czuczwar, S. (2019). Ketogenic Diet in Alzheimer's Disease. *International Journal of Molecular Sciences*, 20. https://doi.org/10.3390/ijms20163892.

[9] Kumar, S., Behl, T., Sachdeva, M., Sehgal, A., Kumari, S., Kumar, A., Kaur, G., Yadav, H., & Bungău, S. (2020). Implicating the effect of ketogenic diet as a preventive measure to obesity and diabetes mellitus.. *Life sciences*, 118661 . https://doi.org/10.1016/j.lfs.2020.118661.

[10] Smyl, C. (2016). Ketogenic Diet and Cancer-a Perspective.. Recent results in cancer research. Fortschritte der Krebsforschung. Progres dans les recherches sur le cancer, 207, 233-40 . https://doi.org/10.1007/978-3-319-42118-6_11.

[11] Kahlon, T. (2006). The new food guide pyramid : Recommendations on grains, fruits, and vegetables. *Cereal Foods World*, 51, 104-107. https://doi.org/10.1094/CFW-51-0104.

[12] Gardner, C., Trepanowski, J., Gobbo, L., Hauser, M., Rigdon, J., Ioannidis, J., Desai, M., & King, A. (2018). Effect of Low-Fat vs Low-Carbohydrate Diet on 12-Month Weight Loss in Overweight Adults and the Association With Genotype Pattern or Insulin Secretion: The DIETFITS Randomized Clinical Trial. *JAMA*, 319, 667–679. https://doi.org/10.1001/jama.2018.0245.

[13] Mayo Clinic Staff (2022). "Carbohydrates: How carbs fit into a healthy diet." *Mayo Clinic*. https://www.mayoclinic.org/healthy-lifestyle/nutrition-and-healthy-eating/in-depth/carbohydrates/art-20045705

[14] Skow, S., & Jha, R. (2022). A Ketogenic Diet is Effective in Improving Insulin Sensitivity in Individuals with Type 2 Diabetes.. *Current diabetes reviews*. https://doi.org/10.2174/1573399818666220425093535.

[15] Chakrabarti, P., & Kandror, K. (2011). Adipose triglyceride lipase: a new target in the regulation of lipolysis by insulin.. *Current diabetes reviews*, 7 4, 270-7 . https://doi.org/10.2174/157339911796397866.

[16] Bebernitz, G., & Schuster, H. (2002). The impact of fatty acid oxidation on energy utilization: targets and therapy.. *Current pharmaceutical design*, 8 14, 1199-227 . https://doi.org/10.2174/1381612023394692.

[17] Schutz, Y. (2011). Protein turnover, ureagenesis and gluconeogenesis.. International journal for vitamin and nutrition research. Internationale Zeitschrift fur Vitamin- und Ernahrungsforschung. Journal international de vitaminologie et de nutrition, 81 2-3, 101-7 . https://doi.org/10.1024/0300-9831/a000064.

[18] Bostock, E., Kirkby, K., Taylor, B., & Hawrelak, J. (2020). Consumer Reports of "Keto Flu" Associated With the Ketogenic Diet. *Frontiers in Nutrition*, 7. https://doi.org/10.3389/fnut.2020.00020.

[19] Wirrell, E. (2008). Ketogenic ratio, calories, and fluids: Do they matter?. *Epilepsia*, 49. https://doi.org/10.1111/j.1528-1167.2008.01825.x.

[20] Bostock, E., Kirkby, K., Taylor, B., & Hawrelak, J. (2020). Consumer Reports of "Keto Flu" Associated With the Ketogenic Diet. *Frontiers in Nutrition*, 7. https://doi.org/10.3389/fnut.2020.00020.

[21] Miller, V., LaFountain, R., Barnhart, E., Sapper, T., Short, J., Arnold, W., Hyde, P., Crabtree, C., Kackley, M., Kraemer, W., Villamena, F., & Volek, J. (2020). A KETOGENIC DIET COMBINED WITH EXERCISE ALTERS MITOCHONDRIAL FUNCTION IN HUMAN SKELETAL MUSCLE WHILE IMPROVING METABOLIC HEALTH.. *American journal of physiology. Endocrinology and metabolism*. https://doi.org/10.1152/ajpendo.00305.2020.

[22] McCarthy, D., & Berg, A. (2021). Weight Loss Strategies and the Risk of Skeletal Muscle Mass Loss. *Nutrients*, 13. https://doi.org/10.3390/nu13072473.

[23] Ashtary-Larky, D., Bagheri, R., Bavi, H., Baker, J., Moro, T., Mancin, L., & Paoli, A. (2021). Ketogenic diets, physical activity and body composition: a review. *The British Journal of Nutrition*, 127, 1898 - 1920. https://doi.org/10.1017/S0007114521002609.